The Other Side of the Vent

The Other Side of the Vent

Helen C. Lee

To order additional copies of this book, contact:
Xlibris Corporation
1-888-795-4274
www.Xlibris.com
Orders@Xlibris.com
77371

Contents

Life is filled with unexpected turns, tumbles, and unexpected changes. These changes can be handled with dignity and grace or with fierce fighting, until you achieve your goals. This year, I and the people in my life were forced into a fierce battle to save my life after becoming a victim of a terrible syndrome called ARDS. ARDS stands for acute respiratory distress syndrome. This syndrome is brought on by an acute serious illness, such as septicemia, from a post-op wound infection, such as I had a post-op hysterectomy. This syndrome takes over the organs and shuts down the organs, including the lungs. With the lungs, the airways become inflamed and the mucus that lines the lungs starts shutting down the bronchial tubes into the lungs and blocks off the alveoli. The alveoli are the sacs at the end of the lungs where oxygen and carbon dioxide are exchanged. Too much carbon dioxide will kill a person, and without clean alveoli, this might happen to me. Without the love, faith, and prayers, I would not be able to write this book. I grew up in a small town in upstate New York called Binghamton. I believe that we have the best health care in this part of the state. We have two major hospitals in this area. I have a wonderful husband, Lance. We have been married for nineteen years and met in a Catholic Singles youth group, and we also met many other friends who married after meeting each other in this group. Lance is a very kind, compassionate, and loving man, who is strong in our faith and has been a wonderful role model of our faith's values to our family and the community. He is giving not only to me, but also to our wonderful son, Matt, and to our Catholic church, the Boy Scouts, and to the Southern tier chapter of the American Red Cross. We have a wonderful son who is also very kind and giving of himself to his friends, church (Matt is an active volunteer for our church's youth group and he is also an altar server), Boy Scouts (he is a Life Scout, which is one step from a Eagle Scout), and he is also a very active volunteer for the Red Cross

The reason I am giving you this background is so you might understand how faith helped us in a chain of events that changed not only how we view how fragile human life is, but also how strong prayers and acts of kindness can impact everyone in your lives. During my nursing career, I treated my patients and their families with kindness, respect, and dignity. I believe that no matter how much education you have and what occupation you're in, that if you treat people with respect and honesty, no matter how long it may take you to deliver a message, people will always think good things about you. This may seem like a simple rule of life, but think of the Golden Rule. Treat people as you would want to be treated in the same situations. This doesn't mean that I have not had difficult situations I had to deal with, but sooner or later, I was able to still help people deal with these situations when they were ready, not when I was ready. This is the basis of part of my book. I found myself ill, and not in control of any part of my body. How I felt how difficult it was for a control freak like myself to give up total control to my health care providers. While you are reading this book, you will see how all these years of nursing and my faith helped me find the way to understand what was happening to me and how this illness affected my family—physically, mentally, and spiritually.

To my husband, Lance; my son, Matthew; the staff of Our Lady of Lourdes Hospital; Drs. Spivak, Fenlon, and Pacheco. Without their expertise, I would not be here today. I would also like to thank my sister, Anne Marie, who could not be with me because she was ill herself, but she was the one who taught me to be stubborn and not give in to anything, even illness and possibly death. Thanks to Anne Marie's husband, Bob, and my niece, Brenna, for their prayers. I would like to thank all of Lance's family, especially Nancy and Jina, for keeping vigil with Lance and I when I was so ill. They were able to keep Lance calm and Matthew happy, when I could not. I would like to thank all of my friends from Seton One and Lourdes at home; Marilyn J., Carol Z., Dana R., Chris K., Patty S., Margo S., Debby N., and all of my United Methodist Homes friends who sat and prayed with myself, Lance, and any other visitors who were in my room; Patty G., Barb R., Tammy J., and Rev. Janet A.

I especially remember these names because they would say the funniest things to me while I was in my worst shape and on the ventilator. These people thought I possibly could hear them. They were correct. I would like to thank all the parishes of St. James, St. Patrick's, the Church of the Holy Family and the many ministers of many faiths, and the wonderful rabbi who came to visit and pray with me. I especially would like to thank Father Ralph from St. James Parish who never missed a day to sit and pray, and when I was able to talk, we talked about food. I would also like to sincerely thank the Daughters of Charity, who also saw me every day and who made sure I received the Body of Christ when I was able to take nourishment. Bless all my family and friends who always made sure that Lance and Matthew were fed; our friends through the running club that Lance belongs to; our friends the Doolittles; Matthew's Scout troupe; the Southern tier chapter of the Red Cross, especially Teresa, Stephanie, and Rebecca; New York State Department of Transportation, whom Lance works for, especially Dave who would come to the hospital on a regular basis to check and see how the whole family was doing; and Lance's good friend at NYSDOT, Linda, who was a great help to Lance during this time. I would also like to thank my longtime friend Steve and his new wife, Johanna, and all of Steve's family—Linda, Dave, Scott, and Keith—who have always treated our family like part of theirs, who also kept Lance and Matthew well fed. Keith even drove in from Buffalo to see me. I always have been known as Aunt Helen to Keith and his brother, Scott, and I have always treated them as nephews.

Chapter One

The Beginning of My Journey

In early December 2008, I developed some irregular bleeding from my female organ; and due to my mother's death in 1998 from ovarian cancer, I immediately made an appointment to see my ob-gyn. My physician suggested I have a pelvic ultrasound to observe and assess whether there was an irregularity in my pelvic region. The test showed a large amount of matter in the uterus. The MD could not make an observation. My physician then scheduled me for a dilatation and curettage of the uterus. This means the physician will go into my uterus and empty its contents, so he is then able to observe and biopsy the tissues in my uterus. This was done two days later, and the MD found a large site that had what appeared to be precancerous cells. The MD did twenty-two biopsies of my uterine tissues, and two days later, the results of the biopsies indicated that I had precancerous cells. The MD talked with me and suggested, due to my mother's history of fast-moving ovarian cancer, we should schedule a complete hysterectomy as soon as possible. After discussions with my husband and other family members, it was decided to do the surgery January 23, 2009. As the days progressed toward the surgical date, I was preparing to be out of commission for at least six weeks. Part of this preparation was to pay bills in advance; to inform Lance, my husband, where my checkbook was, what my cash card code was, where my grocery card is located; and to make amends with anyone whom I had offended in my life. My family couldn't figure why I was doing all these, but my mother had always told me to be prepared for good and bad; that way, you are never taken off guard during an emergency.

I have been a nurse for thirty-three years. For twenty-five years, I had worked as a critical nurse; and the rest of the years, I had worked in home care and a skilled nursing home here in Binghamton, New York, as unit manager. I have a wonderful husband, Lance. We have been married for eighteen years; he is a kind gentleman whom I met at a Catholic Singles youth group. Later in the book, you will see how wonderful Lance really is. We have a wonderful son, Matthew, who is now fifteen and is very active in our community as a volunteer at the Southern chapter of the American Red Cross. He is also a rank of Life Scout in the Boy Scouts of America, and he is in the process of working on his Eagle Scout requirements. In fact, all three of us are very active volunteers with the Red Cross, Boy Scouts, and our church. Matthew is our only son. We had many years of infertility due to my body not cooperating, and when we were able to conceive, we miscarried six children; and at that point, it was time to listen to God and not try anymore. Lance was also the coach of Matthew's school's Odyssey of the Mind team. You can tell we are very busy people and just don't have time to be sick for long, and that is what I was planning on. My plan was just to be out of work for six weeks and then return to normal duties as a nurse.

I am a very positive thinker, and was so when faced with any of the impending surgeries I had, and the outcome had also been positive. I went into surgery that morning with a kiss from my husband, my son, and family—and a prayer in my heart. I am a very strong Catholic. I have always trusted God, and I always have a sense of humor. I believe God has a sense of humor. I returned to my room where my family was waiting for me. I asked what time it was, like almost every patient I have taken care of after a procedure and surgery. I am not quite sure why we ask this question. Maybe there are bettors in any family who would take bets on how long the family member was going to be under anesthesia. No, I am just kidding. I just think we need to know, as patients, how long the surgery was and how long we were in recovery. I can honestly tell you that I and a lot of other people do not remember the answer and will ask this question many times more due to the meds we received in the operating room and recovery room. I continued to ask this question a few more times, and finally, I asked the most important question. Did they get all the precancerous cells out, and did they take a good look around in all my organs to see if anything else was going on in my abdomen? The answer I got was yes, they believe they removed all the problem areas, and they took a good look around and did not see anything suspicious. I asked Lance to call my friends and coworkers and tell them I was doing well, with the pain medicine they were giving me. Later that day, I really woke up and realized I had an IV in my left arm, a tube in my bladder, two long hoses that were connected to special stockings on each leg that alternated external pressure to my legs to prevent blood clots from forming in my legs, because my grandmother in 1954 had died of blood clots, postsurgery of also this type of hysterectomy. I also was connected to oxygen through my nose. And then I realized the pain had started in my abdomen. I realized I was connected to a self-controlling pain med delivery system called a PCA pump. All I had to do is push this little button and a pain med was delivered to me, by way of my IV in my arm; and as I pushed the button, the med worked very quickly, and then I was comfortable again, until they turn me. I learned early to use the pain med before all activity—turning, coughing, and deep breathing. The care I received was excellent from all the staff. During the nurse's assessments every two hours, I had developed a lot of red drainage leaking from my abdominal incision. This was enough to cause concern for the nurse, who added more dressings to my abdomen and applied more direct pressure the dressing, even though I was already wearing a large abdominal binder after surgery. The MD was called at this point. It is now 3:00 a.m. The on-call physician was not my MD, but she was a partner in the group. This MD was at my bedside at six that next morning. This MD was excellent. The MD stated I might be developing a seroma. A seroma is a pocket filled with sterile fluid, drainage, and blood that forms in a cavity where surgery had been performed. Actually, I found out later that this is a very common side effect of this type of surgery, especially when surgery had taken place in the abdomen of a fluffy patient. Use your own definition of *fluffy*. I told you I have a sense of humor.

The wound continued to drain, and a wound culture was taken. That afternoon, my MD who did the surgery arrived in my room and took the dressing down, and the drainage was still quite profuse. My MD stated to me that he felt that I had developed a large seroma, and I would have to have a CT scan to confirm the seroma's presence. The MD released two bottom sutures so that the fluid could drain out of the bottom of the incision. My incision was under the abdominal flap of skin on the lower portion of the abdomen near the bladder. The CT scan was done and confirmed the presence of the seroma. We had a discussion whether I would need a wound VAC placed on the incision. The MD consulted with the local wound care center and other surgeons, and all felt it would be difficult to seal a wound VAC in this area due to my fluffiness. I also agreed that it would be difficult to place this machine on the abdomen and create a tight seal to facilitate the vacuuming of the drainage from the abdomen. We all agreed that we would wait for now for the multiple cultures to come back from the lab. In the meantime, we all discussed that I should be put on a broad-spectrum antibiotic now and to go home on this antibiotic. The multiple cultures came back negative at this time. I was sent home with dressing supplies, and I was taught how to change my dressings at home. The drainage continued at home, but with no change in appearance or odor. I was seeing the surgeon once—and sometimes twice a week; and repeated cultures were done, and no bacteria had grown out. The surgeon suggested I go to our local wound care center that treats difficult wounds with high success rates. The staff at the wound care center were all friends of mine, so I trusted them.

The staff at the wound care center were very helpful, and they repeated another wound culture, and this result came back positive for a very light growth of bacteria. They changed my antibiotic that would have been sensitive to bacteria; we were not happy with the result, but happy we caught it in its early stages. Again a wound VAC was mentioned as a treatment for the wound, but everyone in the wound care center and I felt it would be difficult to place a wound VAC in this area of the abdomen. The wound care center sent me home with a new dressing called Aquacel Ag. For you chemistry buffs, yes, Ag is silver. This dressing inhibits and possibly is antagonistic to bacteria. This treatment was to be packed in my wound as needed, and it would eventually slow the drainage so the wound would need only occasional dressing changes. This dressing was working very well. This drainage was decreasing, and the depth and size of the wound were reducing in size. All of the staff at the wound care center, MDs, nurses, and my family and I were very encouraged by my progress. We are now in the fourth week post-op hysterectomy, and then something changed.

Chapter Two

Something Is Really Wrong

I had been out to dinner with my husband to my all-time favorite Italian restaurant, which is located very close to our home. Our son, Matthew, was on a Boy Scout camping trip at our local Boy Scout Camp. After dinner, I was home, and I stated to Lance that I didn't feel well and something was really wrong. I checked my temperature and found I had a slight fever, 100.4. Normally, my temperature is 97.7. I felt very warm and took some acetaminophen and went to bed. There was no change in discomfort in the abdomen, and there was no change in the drainage, so I decided I would get up again in a few hours to check my temperature. It was 10:30 p.m. I awoke at 2:30 a.m. and really did not feel well, and I was shivering uncontrollably, and my temperature was 104.7. I woke Lance up, and he drove me to my hospital's ER, and I called them ahead of our arrival to give them a report of my condition. Again, I had a sense of humor to call in my own condition en route to the ER, as I had done for many years for my patients. I hit the ER and thanked God it was not busy. After running a few lab tests of blood work and urine, it was determined that I had a urinary tract infection, and my temperature was back down to 98, with acetaminophen and fluids, and that I could go home. I spoke with a friend in the ER (who is one of the nurses I have known for forty years) who stated I could go home, but if I should become worse, I should get right back here and insist on being admitted. I agreed with her opinions, and I agreed to her advice. Lance drove me home. It is now February 22, 2009, at 9:30 a.m. My temperature was normal, and I was going back to bed, and poor Lance had to go to church to pick up Matthew, who was coming back from his camping trip. Lance and Matthew returned home at 12:30 p.m. to find me shivering in my bed; my temperature was 104.7 again, and I was trying to call my attending physician. The physician who was on call for the group called me back and suggested strongly for me to go to the ER again and be admitted directly for evaluation. Lance called his sister, who is a nurse, to oversee Matthew, even though Matt is very mature and is able to stay at home. Matthew stayed home, and Lance drove me to the ER, and my labs were out of control, and I was admitted immediately and started on IVs and IV antibiotics.

I was settled into my hospital bed that was made for fluffy patients, called a bariatric bed. This bed is made to rotate the patient from one side to another and has intermittent air pressure-changing chambers under me so I do not develop bedsores while I was ill. It was Monday morning, February 23, and my wonderful attending physician was standing over my bed when I awoke. Although he was smiling, I could see a concerned look on his face. I noticed I was a little weaker than when I was admitted eight hours ago, and I still had the severe chills, but not as much. He asked me how I felt, and I was honest with him. I admitted that I was not the superhuman *mom* I thought I was and that I thought I must be really septic. A fear ran over my brain. I had cared for many septic patients in my career, and I know that some patients do not do well. But I made myself think, these are more advanced days and new developments are always on the horizon. I trust my physician with my life as I had been with him for fifteen years. My attending informed me that my blood work is a little worse and that I was more short of breath than he would like me to be (I laughed to myself, no shortness of breath would be perfect). He informed me he was going to call in an infection control specialist to help us with my case. I quickly agreed, because she had been a physician my family had known on a professional and a personal level for years.

I was becoming weaker as the day progressed. I was having trouble walking to the bathroom, which was only five feet away from my bed. I was now becoming more short of breath, and my attending physician called in a pulmonologist. Both the infection control and pulmonologist arrived at the same time. They realized that what I had was serious; they started me on new three potent antibiotics and added breathing treatments, and both ordered a battery of blood work and lung scans. At that point, Lance walked in and saw my condition. Lance and the physicians went into the hallway to talk. I knew they were honest with him. My imagination and years of a nurse told me they had probably told him that if I did not improve, I would probably need to go to ICU. As the days progressed, I was feeling a little better, but my blood work had not improved, and a PICC line was put in my arm. A PICC line is a fancy intravenous catheter that is threaded to the upper blood vessel that feeds into my heart so the antibiotics do not damage my arm veins. Thursday morning, a wonderful person came to draw my blood at 600. She had known me for years, and what she found, according to the nurses who were with me, was a very verbally and physically combative person, confused and disoriented. Now, anyone who knows me knew that this was not me. The nurse immediately did vitals and checked my oxygen level, and even with my oxygen in my nose, my oxygen level was extremely low. My attending physician and Lance were called immediately, and both arrived very quickly. My attending MD explained to Lance that my organs were shutting down and my lungs were filling with fluid and I would need to be put into a drug-induced coma and be placed on a ventilator. Throughout all this craziness, Lance was able to keep our friends informed on what my condition was. My friends had been visiting with me the last few days and had also kept Lance up to date, since most of them are health care providers.

Chapter Three

Intensive Care Unit

Once the decision was made to move me to ICU, my attending physician came to my bedside and tried to explain to me that my organs were slowing, shutting down, and he needed to move me quickly. I don't remember much at this point. I do remember having an oxygen mask applied to my face by a respiratory therapist whom I trusted. The look on his face was extremely serious, and he was trying to keep himself and myself calm. I remember a nurse—and I am sorry to say I don't remember her that much—who explained to me that she was going to have to put a catheter in my bladder to drain urine out of me, to keep close track of my intake and output. Another nurse was placing an extra IV in my arm to give me high doses of steroids to decrease the swelling and fluids that were quickly accumulating in my lungs. At this time, even though I was not thinking clearly and the room was starting to spin, I was trying to diagnose myself. *Typical nurse*, I said to myself. I was yelling at myself to quiet my diagnostic mind, but it wasn't working. I thought maybe I had pulmonary emboli (a blood clot to the lung). I was trying to tell the staff that I had a strong family history, on my father's side of the family, of pulmonary emboli, and both family members had this attack at ages between fifty and fifty-three. My age at that time was fifty-three. Then I thought I had pneumonia, but I thought it came on so quickly and with organ failure; it was not pneumonia. At that point, I was telling my mind to trust these friends of mine to save me. I remember having an oxygen tank attached to my bed with my mask on and Lance standing there with my friends and MDs as I was being moved to ICU. I remember the trip to the ICU because we had to go on an elevator, and I remembered to close my eyes in the elevator because I was so dizzy. I remember reaching my ICU room and being met by a group of nurses, some I knew very well and some I didn't know at all. Those nurses were great. They took some time to orient me to what was going on, basically because I was becoming increasingly more anxious. I remember holding Lance's hand and telling him "I love you" over and over. I remember my attending physician and my pulmonary MD standing over me and stating they thought I had a syndrome called ARDS. ARDS is called Acute Respiratory Distress Syndrome. This syndrome is brought on by an acute serious illness, such as septicemia from post op wound infection, such as I had, a post op hysterectomy. This syndrome takes over the organs and shuts down the organs including lungs. With the lungs, the airways become inflamed and the mucus that lines the lungs starts shutting down the bronchial tubes into the lungs and blocks off the alveoli's. The alveoli's are the sacs at the end of the lungs that oxygen and carbon dioxide is exchanged. Too much carbon dioxide will kill a person and without clean alveoli's, this might happen to me. Before I could think straight, the MDs and respiratory therapist inserted an endotracheal tube into my lungs and hooked me to a ventilator after I was sedated.

Lessons these experiences taught me and which I want to share with others are many. When my friends and I were in nursing schools and health-related schools, we learned that hearing is the last sense to go before people die. We were taught to always to talk to our patients and families when we are giving care. I can honestly tell you this is a huge issue to cover. I can tell you who came into my room. I can tell you, sometimes very accurately and sometimes not, what people in the room said or the general idea of the conversation. I don't know exactly what day this episode happened, but it happened, and I will describe it in graphic detail. I could feel myself flying. I know I was in a drug-induced coma for nine days, and I know this could have given the experience of flying. I remember flying, and then I saw this bright light in front of me. I remember thinking the old saying, "Don't go near the light." I remember thinking that light was so bright, and very quickly, clear vision took over, and I could see my late mother and father; mother-in-law; my infant niece, who was shown as a teenager (which is what she would have been if she were alive); my adult niece, whom we had lost to cancer. I also saw a young man, whom I knew was my friend's son, who had drowned when he was little. Circling them were six floating bright forms that I knew were our six children we had lost in miscarriages. I remember my father looking at me with a very curious look on his face—and if anyone knows someone Italian, and you know Italians, we talk with our hands and arms—he gave me the gesture of *why are you here?* He then waved me off, and I floated back into my bed. I remember waking to the sound of my pulmonologist's wonderful voice trying to arouse me. I had tears in my eyes, and he wiped my tears away and told me he was working hard to stabilize me and to be patient with him. I can remember the nurses who immediately entered the room at this time. They were getting ready to turn me when I heard one nurse say to the other nurse, "I am not sure she is going to make it. She is not in good shape at this time, and we can't keep her blood pressure up. Her organs are not responding to the steroids." Now, I heard just enough, plus I had just gone through the flying experience, and I thought to myself, *I will show you guys. I am a tough, stubborn Italian Irish mom, nurse, and a wife to a wonderful man, and I am going to make it.* At that moment, I made myself more in tune to what was going on around me, or maybe the MDs and nurses had backed off on the sedation, but I knew I was going to make it.

All right, we need some of my humorous moments in this book, and I have a lot of them to share. I am sharing them to show that health care without some humor is just too stressful on everyone. Again, I want to emphasize that hearing is very present to people even in a drug-induced coma. When I was not stable, especially the first four days in ICU, many of my health care friends and family stayed with Lance in the ICU. I can remember my friend Marilyn coming into my room and shouting, "Hey, what are you doing in that bed? We have to get you better and get you out of here. I can't shove a Panera Bread sandwich down your feeding tube. Maybe the soup, but definitely not the bread bowl." I remember people laughing in the room. I remember trying to laugh, but I was so deep in sedation, my body wasn't cooperating to laugh. I remember Marilyn talking to me, telling me this was not the place for me. I needed to be out working on the other side of the bed, like I used to do. Many discussions from many of my *friends* talked of how we had run codes and saved people's lives together and that there were more people out there who needed my help. My sister-in-law, Jina, brought in a radio with a CD player. Lance had brought in my favorite contemporary Christian rock CDs. I remember the day they set up the radio in my room. Even though I could not respond outward to this music, inside I was less stressed-out, much calmer, more at peace with the surroundings. The music both from the radio and my CDs lessened the stress for my family and friends. I found, with the music, there was a more relaxed and positive speaking in the room by all. I found myself trying to be more attentive to the music and the news that I was listening to. I found that certain songs reminded me what a wonderful family and friends I had and what a wonderful life I had, up until this point, and would continue for many years to come. The music gave me courage that I was being cared for by my friends and that I was going to make it. I was not aware I was on a ventilator, because of the sedation, until the last three days on the ventilator, which is probably a good thing. I can remember my friends keeping vigil at the bedside with Lance and my other family members. I can remember many visits with my friends, and they were making jokes—how I lost weight, but that it was the wrong way to do it. I had to laugh to myself that the topic was always food, nursing, prayer, and *Star Trek*. My friends and I had gone through some very difficult times, both in nursing and our private lives, by quoting our favorite *Star Trek* sayings such as "Darn it, Jim, I am a doctor, not a scientist." My friends always made sure that Lance was eating and trying to get rest. They were always trying to get Lance out of the room, so he could not get sick himself. My friends were always talking with Lance about what they were going to make for my family to eat. I can remember quite a few days when my friends would come in and say the rosary with me. And I used my fingers to count off the prayers so I could also feel the prayers, not just hear the prayers. I can remember at times my family and friends, putting my CDs in and holding my hands. Some visitors were in my room so often, they became aware of the songs and would sing them. My family and friends all knew I was a decent singer, so they made sure when a song came on, they would sing with the song, knowing that if I could, I would be singing with them. I remember one day when a group of nurses were in my room, giving care to me, singing very loudly to me, "There ain't no mountain high enough." Inside, I thought, *What an appropriate song for me.* God bless them. I can remember the day there was a commotion in the ICU. All I could hear was a lot of activity. Before I knew it, my friend Marylyn ran into my room and, in a loud voice, said, "Thank God it is not you," and ran out. I found out a week later there was a CPR in the ICU that day, and my friends were worried it was me. I have a special woman in my life. Her name is Mrs. K. She was my mother's best friend. She and her husband had many children, and to this day, her family is still very close to our family. This wonderful woman lived down the street when we were growing up. When my mother died, Mrs. K. took over the role of my mother. Mrs. K. was there every day. She questioned everything the ICU nurses did for me. Thank God when I initially was admitted to the hospital, we had put her on the list to give information to. I knew if I did not do that, she would be miserable. Mrs. K. directed the traffic in my room. She made sure that Lance did not get overtired. She made sure my visitors did not stay too long to tire myself and Lance out. She made sure I was getting the best care all the time, which I was. She would sit at my bedside, praying the rosary and novenas. She would make sure that my radio was turned on. She announced my visitors, talked with my family and friends, and tried to keep the noise level down, even though I loved hearing voices. Anyone who knows me knows that I love joyful noise. I would not trade her for the world. The major role she had if a new person came into my room would be to ask for their job title and how long they had been doing their job and had they worked with this type of patient before. God love her.

The nurses I had were excellent. They would tell me everything they were doing. Many nurses who took care of me, I had worked with for many years. This made me feel secure in my care. In fact, it must have been difficult to take care of one of their friends and ex-coworkers. Some of these nurses I actually helped orient in their nursing roles. Trust and calmness were always in place for me. There was not a moment I felt uncared for. The staff and MDs were wonderful to explain everything to Lance and my family. I started feeling a little more attentive as the days progressed. I found out later, as I was becoming more stable, the staff was able to lighten my sedation, when Lance and the MDs were in the room, so I could be more aware of my disease and prognosis. The best few days were approximately three days before the tube was taken out of my lungs. During these days, the nurses were reducing my sedation so I could try to get off the ventilator. The first few days, I was too weak, and I could not breathe without the help of the ventilator. Finally, the day arrived when the MDs and respiratory therapists agreed that I had showed improvement, and my arterial blood gasses were stable. I can remember my attending physician and pulmonologist telling me they were going to take the tube out of my lungs. This was, and I knew it, a monumental day. My attending stated, "Do not hit your physician when the tube comes out, and do not yell at your physicians. Remember, the MDs and nurses saved your life."

The tube is out, I can speak again, I was thinking. But nine days on the ventilator had left me with a whispery voice. *Oh, this is just great. I had a million questions, and I can't even talk,* I thought to myself. I knew this was normal, and it would take time to have my voice return to normal. Just then, Lance walked into the room, and we cried and held each other tight, and then cried some more, and I whispered many times over and over that I loved him, and a million times more, he repeated "I love you." The room was a mess; MDs, nurses, and respiratory therapists were all crying. When I think about it, what a celebration of life.

Chapter Four

And Now the Fun Begins

W hen the dust settled, a nurse came in with oral care supplies. Even though the nurses were giving me oral care all the time, there is nothing like brushing your teeth. The shock then hit me: because of the disease syndrome, it had left me with the inability to move my hands or arms to pick up a toothbrush or a cup of ice or anything. The nurse stated this was normal due to my extensive illness, and she would help me with my teeth and with the ice chips. I started crying again, and this time not for joy. I whispered, "I want to see an occupational therapist now." The nurse was kind and gentle and stated she would contact them as soon as possible. I knew this sometimes happens with really ill patients, but I was a busy woman, and I was not going to be a burden to anyone. The occupational therapist came to visit me. She informed me that due to long-term sedation—and I now had noticed my extremely swollen hands—from the steroids, that I would get the movement back. She gave me some wonderful exercises to do to strengthen my hands and arms. With much frustration and tears, I had gross motor movement back in my arms and hands by day 4 off the ventilator. This meant I could finally feed myself without putting pudding and ice chips in my hair. I felt sorry for Lance because I wanted to feed myself in the beginning, and he saw many ice chips and pudding land in areas they were not intended to land. Lance and I mentioned that someday we will laugh about my lack of aim, and now at the writing of the book, I can laugh at this point in the recovery. We let our son visit me since I was off the ventilator. What a wonderful sight to see his *mom* looking fair. We were all smiling so much, we should have hooked up solar panels to collect the radiation. Matt was relieved I was progressing. Lance and my family did a wonderful job prepping Matt to see me. I still had IVs and a wound VAC and a catheter in my bladder, but the nurses did a wonderful job to hide these tubes. My friends and family all got the word I was off the tube, both the breathing tube and the tube feeding in my stomach. My friends were rejoicing. Two days after coming off the ventilator, I was moved to a step-down unit with a wonderful staff. I was moved late in the evening, the night before the Odyssey of the Mind competition, and Lance was concerned about my being on a regular unit and him being in an all-day competition with Matthew and his team. Friends heard about this situation and took shifts sitting with me so that Lance could feel secure to be away from me. Mrs. K. was with me when I was moved out of ICU and asked many questions and made sure that she was comfortable with me being out of ICU. After I was settled in my new bed, and after she was secure with leaving me on this unit, Mrs. K. went home to return bright and early. She wanted to make sure I was being cared for properly. I and Mrs. K. were very happy with the care I was receiving. Matt and his team came in third in his division. That evening, Matt and Lance appeared in my room, looking very tired but very happy. They brought me the trophy, and Lance had videoed the whole competition and award ceremony, and I watched every second of it. I was so proud of them and the team. I don't know how Lance kept his sanity during this whole time of preparing the team for the competition and still have Matt active with Scouting, and my illness. All of our friends from all of our contacts with the community and family kept on top of Matt and Lance. They continued to prepare food and anything else the guys needed, including financial aid. This was a difficult time financially, with this recovery taking a lot longer than I and Lance ever suspected. But thanks to the generosity of our family and friends, Lance was able to be creative with our finances.

I cannot thank enough the physical therapists, occupational therapists, and speech therapists for being persistent and encouraging in my recovery. As I mentioned before, when I was taken off the ventilator, I realized I could not feed myself or take care of any of my personal needs. All the therapy departments gave a full-court press. It helped that many of them knew me at prior baseline and where we had to go; I had to go to a rehabilitation unit for at least two weeks. My plan was set by myself and the physical and occupational therapists on a daily basis. There were a lot of days that I wanted to do more than the therapists thought I could accomplish. I was so stubborn—and I had a serious, maybe not a rational, sense of humor—that the therapists and aides let me try to accomplish my goals. My goals did not go well the first four days. I had now regained my gross motor skills so that, with assistance, I was able to almost feed myself. It took many days of attempting to at least keep my balance sitting on the edge of the bed. Then on day 4, I told everyone I was going to walk to the chair and sit in the chair for a short period. The therapists were thrilled that I felt that strong. There I was, finally ready to stand and take my steps, when some wonderful nurse and physical therapist friends came into the room. I knew I had three physical therapists, two nurses, and two aides in my room, all giving me directions. I realized something very quickly. I realized that any patient, young or old, becomes confused and agitated when there is too much commotion and people in the room giving directions. Now, don't get me wrong. I would never trade any of them in for new friends, but I finally asked if one person could give directions. At this point, myself and everyone in the room started laughing, and everyone took the situation as a positive learning experience. I was able to walk a few feet and sit in the chair. I have never seen people laugh, cry, and rejoice as I did that. That went better than everyone expected, but the next hurdle was if I could stand from a chair and walk back to my bed. I tried much faster than I expected, and I was helped back to the bed before I became totally fatigued. The initial stand was tough, but I was able to return to my bed. The really glorious day was when I walked twenty feet to the bathroom and was able to use the facilities. I insisted that they take the tube out of my bladder the next day, which would make me walk more to the bathroom. Every day, I walked much longer in the hallway with assistance from the staff, and I progressed so quickly I bypassed the discharge goals at the rehab center where I would have gone to for extensive rehab therapy. Hurray! I was told I could go home, but there was still a major hurdle that I had not addressed in this book yet. The problem is that, for some reason, my potassium and magnesium would not stay in my system. Almost every day, the nurses had to infuse me with large doses of potassium and magnesium through my IV. Finally, after many days and also working with the dietitian, myself and my wonderful primary physician realized that during my multiorgan shutdown, my kidney had been damaged and could not retain the potassium and magnesium. My physician put me on potassium-sparing meds that were able to keep my electrolytes in order. Finally, when all my issues were stable, the plan was put into place to go home. I still needed a VAC attached to my abdomen. Because of the VAC, I would need a nurse to come to my house three times a week to change my dressing. Because I was still quite weak in walking and personal care, we also decided to send me home with physical therapist and occupational therapist visits to get me stronger and, eventually, get me off the walker; and when the wound healed, I could be stable to shower. With most delay because of insurance and VAC availability, I was able to be discharged to my home, with my husband and son. That was a marvelous day. With much assistance as I walked in the living room, there was my son, Matt, and he had made the biggest welcome-home banner for me. He prominently hung the banner across my large picture windows so I could see it as I walked in the living room. We cried of joy. The next day, my home care nurse, Nellie, came to admit me to the home care services. It felt very weird to be on the other side of the bed again, since I used to be a home care nurse. Nellie was wonderful. She was kind and very supportive throughout the very long recovery at home. Nellie was very efficient, and I wanted nothing more. She reminded me of what I was like when I was younger. She had a terrific sense of humor, and as you know, I needed that to recover. It took a very long time for my wound to heal and to get the VAC off my abdomen. It looked like a very stylish purse. I had not worn a purse for about fifteen years since before I had Matt. Once the wound VAC was taken off, it took a while to heal. But Nellie still had a terrific sense of humor, and she was very intelligent with how she handled my case. Throughout this care at home, I received many hours of therapy from Bill. Bill stood about six feet four inches and was a gentle giant who had me do activities I never did or could do before my illness. Before I knew it, he had me off the walker and walking slowly up and down the stairs and working on my exercise machine and walking up and down my steep road. The exercises he gave me to do were centered on core and extremity strengthening. I slowly but steadily became more confident and steady on my feet. The day he discharged me was a bittersweet day, because he had the sense of humor that actually encouraged me and made me want to do exercises after I got better. Was that me thinking those thoughts? Finally, the day had come when the wound had healed, and Nellie discharged me from the service. Also, that was another bittersweet day. Nellie was able to keep my sense of humor going in a very long and scary time at home. God bless this home care agency and its wonderful caregivers.

Chapter Five

Back to Work

The day has come for me to have my wound evaluated by my primary physician and to receive his final approval to send me back to work. Throughout this ordeal, my physician and his office have been extremely supportive but cautious on when I could go back to work. It was January 23, the initial surgery, and it is now May 28. I informed the physician that I wanted and needed to go back full time. He, in his kind and caring manner, informed me he will send me back part time for ten days, and then if I feel well enough, I can return to full time. I reluctantly agreed with him, and I will comply; after all, he and the talented team of other physicians and nurses saved my life. Who am I to go against his decision? Is that me talking? I informed my wonderful employer, who saved my job for me, that I would be returning. There was much rejoicing—by my family, all of my friends from all walks of life, and my employer—that I am now starting a new chapter (literally) in my life.

Chapter Six

What I Have Learned or Relearned

I want to emphasize that every day is a miracle that we are alive. We should never take these days for granted. Never take our family or families for granted. We should always—and I know this can be difficult, but you should—be involved in our community activities. Open yourself up to new life experiences. Don't waste your life and talents. Everyone has talents. It's what you do with God's present of your talents that makes you the person you are. Try to have a sense of humor when things go bad in your life. A positive thinker will help you through many challenges through your life. Try to love and respect all the people you are in contact with. I know this is also difficult, but try. Your positive influence may change another person's perception of life. This might help change that person's life for the better. Love your family, friends, and coworkers with all your heart. Your love will shine through, and they just might need that positive moment some day. When you run into a difficult person, take the time to listen to that person. That person may have a point to make and may just need someone to help put the concern into perspective to help them really look at the reason they are feeling or acting difficult that day. Life changes in a matter of minutes. Be open in your mind, body, and spirit to cope with this life-changing experience. Is this tough? Oh yes, it most certainly is. I never thought my life would change in minutes, or my family would be tested and stressed in all different directions, or my friends would be faced with the serious illness of one of their friends. We all deal with illness in a different manner. I just happened to be blessed with the satisfaction that I survived only by the grace of God, who was able to support and guide my physicians, caregivers, friends, family, and especially Lance and Matt through these troubled waters. Without prayers from everyone, I would not have been able to write this book.

www.ingramcontent.com/pod-product-compliance
Lightning Source LLC
Chambersburg PA
CBHW050345290526
45785CB00006B/2645